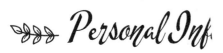 *Personal Info*

NAME : _____

ADRESS : _____

_____

PHONE : _____

EMAIL : _____

MEDICATIONS : _____

BLOOD TYPE : _____

ALLERGIES : _____

Insurance Information

CARRIER : _____

POLICY # : _____

PHONE : _____

Emergency Contact

NAME : _____

PHONE : _____

RELATIONSHIP : _____

DATE : _____   S   M   T   W   T   F   S

Today Goals

_____

_____

_____

_____

_____

_____

Mood

○ Happy   ○ Stressed

○ Relaxed   ○ Anxious

○ Tired   ○ Sad

○ Inspired   ○ Angry

Energy Level

○   ○   ○
Low   Med   High

Blood Sugar & Food Tracker

Time/Meal	Blood Sugar Levels		Foods
	Before	After	
Wake-up Reading			
Breakfast			
Lunch			
Dinner			
Snacks			
Bedtime Reading			

Meds / Supplements

Water Intake

Activity

Sleep

Daily Schedule

Time	
5:00	
6:00	
7:00	
8:00	
9:00	
10:00	
11:00	
12:00	
13:00	
14:00	
15:00	
16:00	
17:00	
18:00	
19:00	
20:00	
21:00	
22:00	
23:00	

Notes: _____
_____
_____
_____
_____

DATE: _____   S   M   T   W   T   F   S

Today Goals

_____
_____
_____
_____
_____
_____

Mood

○ Happy   ○ Stressed
○ Relaxed   ○ Anxious
○ Tired   ○ Sad
○ Inspired   ○ Angry

Energy Level

○   ○   ○
Low   Med   High

Blood Sugar & Food Tracker

Time/Meal	Blood Sugar Levels		Foods
	Before	After	
Wake-up Reading			
Breakfast			
Lunch			
Dinner			
Snacks			
Bedtime Reading			

Meds / Supplements

Water Intake

Activity

Sleep

Daily Schedule

5:00	
6:00	
7:00	
8:00	
9:00	
10:00	
11:00	
12:00	
13:00	
14:00	
15:00	
16:00	
17:00	
18:00	
19:00	
20:00	
21:00	
22:00	
23:00	

Notes:

DATE: _____   S M T W T F S

Today Goals

_____
_____
_____
_____
_____

Mood

○ Happy   ○ Stressed
○ Relaxed   ○ Anxious
○ Tired   ○ Sad
○ Inspired   ○ Angry

Energy Level

○   ○   ○
Low   Med   High

Blood Sugar & Food Tracker

Time/Meal	Blood Sugar Levels		Foods
	Before	After	
Wake-up Reading			
Breakfast			
Lunch			
Dinner			
Snacks			
Bedtime Reading			

Meds / Supplements

Water Intake

Activity

Sleep

Daily Schedule

5:00	
6:00	
7:00	
8:00	
9:00	
10:00	
11:00	
12:00	
13:00	
14:00	
15:00	
16:00	
17:00	
18:00	
19:00	
20:00	
21:00	
22:00	
23:00	

Notes: _____

_____

_____

_____

_____

DATE: _____   S M T W T F S

Today Goals

_____
_____
_____
_____
_____
_____

Mood

○ Happy   ○ Stressed
○ Relaxed   ○ Anxious
○ Tired   ○ Sad
○ Inspired   ○ Angry

Energy Level

○ Low   ○ Med   ○ High

Blood Sugar & Food Tracker

Time/Meal	Blood Sugar Levels		Foods
	Before	After	
Wake-up Reading			
Breakfast			
Lunch			
Dinner			
Snacks			
Bedtime Reading			

Meds / Supplements

Water Intake

Activity

Sleep

Daily Schedule

Time	
5:00	
6:00	
7:00	
8:00	
9:00	
10:00	
11:00	
12:00	
13:00	
14:00	
15:00	
16:00	
17:00	
18:00	
19:00	
20:00	
21:00	
22:00	
23:00	

Notes: _____
_____
_____
_____
_____

DATE : _____   S M T W T F S

Today Goals

_____
_____
_____
_____
_____
_____

Mood

- ○ Happy
- ○ Relaxed
- ○ Tired
- ○ Inspired
- ○ Stressed
- ○ Anxious
- ○ Sad
- ○ Angry

Energy Level

○   ○   ○
Low   Med   High

Blood Sugar & Food Tracker

Time/Meal	Blood Sugar Levels		Foods
	Before	After	
Wake-up Reading			
Breakfast			
Lunch			
Dinner			
Snacks			
Bedtime Reading			

Meds / Supplements

Water Intake

Activity

Sleep

Daily Schedule

5:00	
6:00	
7:00	
8:00	
9:00	
10:00	
11:00	
12:00	
13:00	
14:00	
15:00	
16:00	
17:00	
18:00	
19:00	
20:00	
21:00	
22:00	
23:00	

Notes:

DATE: _____   S   M   T   W   T   F   S

Today Goals

_____
_____
_____
_____
_____
_____

Mood

○ Happy   ○ Stressed
○ Relaxed   ○ Anxious
○ Tired   ○ Sad
○ Inspired   ○ Angry

Energy Level

○   ○   ○
Low   Med   High

Blood Sugar & Food Tracker

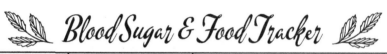

Time/Meal	Blood Sugar Levels		Foods
	Before	After	
Wake-up Reading			
Breakfast			
Lunch			
Dinner			
Snacks			
Bedtime Reading			

Meds / Supplements

Water Intake

Activity

Sleep

Daily Schedule

Time	
5:00	
6:00	
7:00	
8:00	
9:00	
10:00	
11:00	
12:00	
13:00	
14:00	
15:00	
16:00	
17:00	
18:00	
19:00	
20:00	
21:00	
22:00	
23:00	

Notes:

DATE: _____   S   M   T   W   T   F   S

Today Goals

_____

_____

_____

_____

_____

_____

Mood

- ○ Happy
- ○ Relaxed
- ○ Tired
- ○ Inspired

- ○ Stressed
- ○ Anxious
- ○ Sad
- ○ Angry

Energy Level

○   ○   ○
Low   Med   High

Blood Sugar & Food Tracker

Time/Meal	Blood Sugar Levels		Foods
	Before	After	
Wake-up Reading			
Breakfast			
Lunch			
Dinner			
Snacks			
Bedtime Reading			

Meds / Supplements

Water Intake

Activity

Sleep

Daily Schedule

5:00	
6:00	
7:00	
8:00	
9:00	
10:00	
11:00	
12:00	
13:00	
14:00	
15:00	
16:00	
17:00	
18:00	
19:00	
20:00	
21:00	
22:00	
23:00	

Notes: _____
_____
_____
_____
_____

DATE: _____   S M T W T F S

Today Goals

_____
_____
_____
_____
_____
_____

Mood

○ Happy   ○ Stressed
○ Relaxed   ○ Anxious
○ Tired   ○ Sad
○ Inspired   ○ Angry

Energy Level

○   ○   ○
Low   Med   High

Blood Sugar & Food Tracker

Time/Meal	Blood Sugar Levels		Foods
	Before	After	
Wake-up Reading			
Breakfast			
Lunch			
Dinner			
Snacks			
Bedtime Reading			

Meds / Supplements

Water Intake

Activity

Sleep

Daily Schedule

Time	
5:00	
6:00	
7:00	
8:00	
9:00	
10:00	
11:00	
12:00	
13:00	
14:00	
15:00	
16:00	
17:00	
18:00	
19:00	
20:00	
21:00	
22:00	
23:00	

Notes:

DATE: _____   S   M   T   W   T   F   S

Today Goals

_____
_____
_____
_____
_____
_____

Mood

○ Happy   ○ Stressed
○ Relaxed   ○ Anxious
○ Tired   ○ Sad
○ Inspired   ○ Angry

Energy Level

○   ○   ○
Low   Med   High

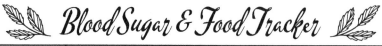

Blood Sugar & Food Tracker

Time/Meal	Blood Sugar Levels		Foods
	Before	After	
Wake-up Reading			
Breakfast			
Lunch			
Dinner			
Snacks			
Bedtime Reading			

— Meds / Supplements —

— Water Intake —

Activity

Sleep

⚘ Daily Schedule ⚘

5:00	
6:00	
7:00	
8:00	
9:00	
10:00	
11:00	
12:00	
13:00	
14:00	
15:00	
16:00	
17:00	
18:00	
19:00	
20:00	
21:00	
22:00	
23:00	

Notes:

DATE: _____   S M T W T F S

Today Goals

_____
_____
_____
_____
_____
_____

Mood

○ Happy   ○ Stressed
○ Relaxed   ○ Anxious
○ Tired   ○ Sad
○ Inspired   ○ Angry

Energy Level

○   ○   ○
Low   Med   High

Blood Sugar & Food Tracker

Time/Meal	Blood Sugar Levels		Foods
	Before	After	
Wake-up Reading			
Breakfast			
Lunch			
Dinner			
Snacks			
Bedtime Reading			

Meds / Supplements

Water Intake

Activity

Sleep

Daily Schedule

Time	
5:00	
6:00	
7:00	
8:00	
9:00	
10:00	
11:00	
12:00	
13:00	
14:00	
15:00	
16:00	
17:00	
18:00	
19:00	
20:00	
21:00	
22:00	
23:00	

Notes: _____

_____

_____

_____

_____

DATE: _____   S   M   T   W   T   F   S

Today Goals

_____
_____
_____
_____
_____
_____

Mood

○ Happy   ○ Stressed
○ Relaxed   ○ Anxious
○ Tired   ○ Sad
○ Inspired   ○ Angry

Energy Level

○   ○   ○
Low   Med   High

Blood Sugar & Food Tracker

Time/Meal	Blood Sugar Levels		Foods
	Before	After	
Wake-up Reading			
Breakfast			
Lunch			
Dinner			
Snacks			
Bedtime Reading			

Meds / Supplements

Water Intake

Activity

Sleep

Daily Schedule

Time	
5:00	
6:00	
7:00	
8:00	
9:00	
10:00	
11:00	
12:00	
13:00	
14:00	
15:00	
16:00	
17:00	
18:00	
19:00	
20:00	
21:00	
22:00	
23:00	

Notes: _____

DATE: _____   S   M   T   W   T   F   S

Today Goals

_____

_____

_____

_____

_____

_____

Mood

○ Happy   ○ Stressed
○ Relaxed   ○ Anxious
○ Tired   ○ Sad
○ Inspired   ○ Angry

Energy Level

○   ○   ○
Low   Med   High

Blood Sugar & Food Tracker

Time/Meal	Blood Sugar Levels		Foods
	Before	After	
Wake-up Reading			
Breakfast			
Lunch			
Dinner			
Snacks			
Bedtime Reading			

— Meds/Supplements —

— Water Intake —

— Activity —

— Sleep —

Daily Schedule

Time	
5:00	
6:00	
7:00	
8:00	
9:00	
10:00	
11:00	
12:00	
13:00	
14:00	
15:00	
16:00	
17:00	
18:00	
19:00	
20:00	
21:00	
22:00	
23:00	

Notes:

DATE: _____   S   M   T   W   T   F   S

Today Goals

_____

_____

_____

_____

_____

_____

Mood

- ○ Happy   ○ Stressed
- ○ Relaxed   ○ Anxious
- ○ Tired   ○ Sad
- ○ Inspired   ○ Angry

Energy Level

○	○	○
Low	Med	High

Blood Sugar & Food Tracker

Time/Meal	Blood Sugar Levels		Foods
	Before	After	
Wake-up Reading			
Breakfast			
Lunch			
Dinner			
Snacks			
Bedtime Reading			

Meds / Supplements

Water Intake

Activity

Sleep

Daily Schedule

5:00	
6:00	
7:00	
8:00	
9:00	
10:00	
11:00	
12:00	
13:00	
14:00	
15:00	
16:00	
17:00	
18:00	
19:00	
20:00	
21:00	
22:00	
23:00	

Notes: _____

DATE: _____   S M T W T F S

Today Goals

_____
_____
_____
_____
_____
_____

Mood

○ Happy   ○ Stressed
○ Relaxed   ○ Anxious
○ Tired   ○ Sad
○ Inspired   ○ Angry

Energy Level

○   ○   ○
Low   Med   High

Blood Sugar & Food Tracker

Time/Meal	Blood Sugar Levels		Foods
	Before	After	
Wake-up Reading			
Breakfast			
Lunch			
Dinner			
Snacks			
Bedtime Reading			

Meds / Supplements

Water Intake

Activity

Sleep

Daily Schedule

Time	
5:00	
6:00	
7:00	
8:00	
9:00	
10:00	
11:00	
12:00	
13:00	
14:00	
15:00	
16:00	
17:00	
18:00	
19:00	
20:00	
21:00	
22:00	
23:00	

Notes: _____

DATE : _____   S   M   T   W   T   F   S

Today Goals

_____
_____
_____
_____
_____
_____

Mood

○ Happy   ○ Stressed
○ Relaxed   ○ Anxious
○ Tired   ○ Sad
○ Inspired   ○ Angry

Energy Level

○   ○   ○
Low   Med   High

Blood Sugar & Food Tracker

Time/Meal	Blood Sugar Levels		Foods
	Before	After	
Wake-up Reading			
Breakfast			
Lunch			
Dinner			
Snacks			
Bedtime Reading			

— Meds/Supplements —

— Water Intake —

— Activity —

— Sleep —

Daily Schedule

Time	
5:00	
6:00	
7:00	
8:00	
9:00	
10:00	
11:00	
12:00	
13:00	
14:00	
15:00	
16:00	
17:00	
18:00	
19:00	
20:00	
21:00	
22:00	
23:00	

Notes:

DATE: _____   S M T W T F S

Today Goals

_____
_____
_____
_____
_____
_____

Mood

○ Happy   ○ Stressed
○ Relaxed   ○ Anxious
○ Tired   ○ Sad
○ Inspired   ○ Angry

Energy Level

○ Low   ○ Med   ○ High

Blood Sugar & Food Tracker

Time/Meal	Blood Sugar Levels		Foods
	Before	After	
Wake-up Reading			
Breakfast			
Lunch			
Dinner			
Snacks			
Bedtime Reading			

Meds / Supplements

Water Intake

Activity

Sleep

Daily Schedule

Time	
5:00	
6:00	
7:00	
8:00	
9:00	
10:00	
11:00	
12:00	
13:00	
14:00	
15:00	
16:00	
17:00	
18:00	
19:00	
20:00	
21:00	
22:00	
23:00	

Notes: _____
_____
_____
_____
_____

DATE: _____   S M T W T F S

Today Goals

_____
_____
_____
_____
_____
_____

Mood

○ Happy   ○ Stressed
○ Relaxed   ○ Anxious
○ Tired   ○ Sad
○ Inspired   ○ Angry

Energy Level

○   ○   ○
Low   Med   High

Blood Sugar & Food Tracker

Time/Meal	Blood Sugar Levels		Foods
	Before	After	
Wake-up Reading			
Breakfast			
Lunch			
Dinner			
Snacks			
Bedtime Reading			

Meds / Supplements

Water Intake

Activity

Sleep

Daily Schedule

5:00	
6:00	
7:00	
8:00	
9:00	
10:00	
11:00	
12:00	
13:00	
14:00	
15:00	
16:00	
17:00	
18:00	
19:00	
20:00	
21:00	
22:00	
23:00	

Notes:

DATE : _____   S   M   T   W   T   F   S

Today Goals

_____
_____
_____
_____
_____
_____

Mood

○ Happy   ○ Stressed
○ Relaxed   ○ Anxious
○ Tired   ○ Sad
○ Inspired   ○ Angry

Energy Level

○   ○   ○
Low   Med   High

Blood Sugar & Food Tracker

Time/Meal	Blood Sugar Levels		Foods
	Before	After	
Wake-up Reading			
Breakfast			
Lunch			
Dinner			
Snacks			
Bedtime Reading			

Meds / Supplements

Water Intake

Activity

Sleep

Daily Schedule

5:00	
6:00	
7:00	
8:00	
9:00	
10:00	
11:00	
12:00	
13:00	
14:00	
15:00	
16:00	
17:00	
18:00	
19:00	
20:00	
21:00	
22:00	
23:00	

Notes:

DATE: _____   S   M   T   W   T   F   S

Today Goals

_____
_____
_____
_____
_____
_____

Mood

○ Happy   ○ Stressed
○ Relaxed   ○ Anxious
○ Tired   ○ Sad
○ Inspired   ○ Angry

Energy Level

○   ○   ○
Low   Med   High

Blood Sugar & Food Tracker

Time/Meal	Blood Sugar Levels		Foods
	Before	After	
Wake-up Reading			
Breakfast			
Lunch			
Dinner			
Snacks			
Bedtime Reading			

Meds / Supplements

Water Intake

Activity

Sleep

Daily Schedule

Time	
5:00	
6:00	
7:00	
8:00	
9:00	
10:00	
11:00	
12:00	
13:00	
14:00	
15:00	
16:00	
17:00	
18:00	
19:00	
20:00	
21:00	
22:00	
23:00	

Notes:

DATE: _____   S M T W T F S

Today Goals

_____

_____

_____

_____

_____

_____

Mood

○ Happy   ○ Stressed

○ Relaxed   ○ Anxious

○ Tired   ○ Sad

○ Inspired   ○ Angry

Energy Level

○   ○   ○

Low   Med   High

Blood Sugar & Food Tracker

Time/Meal	Blood Sugar Levels		Foods
	Before	After	
Wake-up Reading			
Breakfast			
Lunch			
Dinner			
Snacks			
Bedtime Reading			

Meds / Supplements

Water Intake

Activity

Sleep

Daily Schedule

Time	
5:00	
6:00	
7:00	
8:00	
9:00	
10:00	
11:00	
12:00	
13:00	
14:00	
15:00	
16:00	
17:00	
18:00	
19:00	
20:00	
21:00	
22:00	
23:00	

Notes:

DATE : _____   S M T W T F S

Today Goals

_____
_____
_____
_____
_____
_____

Mood

○ Happy   ○ Stressed
○ Relaxed   ○ Anxious
○ Tired   ○ Sad
○ Inspired   ○ Angry

Energy Level

○ Low   ○ Med   ○ High

Blood Sugar & Food Tracker

Time/Meal	Blood Sugar Levels		Foods
	Before	After	
Wake-up Reading			
Breakfast			
Lunch			
Dinner			
Snacks			
Bedtime Reading			

Meds / Supplements

Water Intake

Activity

Sleep

Daily Schedule

Time	
5:00	
6:00	
7:00	
8:00	
9:00	
10:00	
11:00	
12:00	
13:00	
14:00	
15:00	
16:00	
17:00	
18:00	
19:00	
20:00	
21:00	
22:00	
23:00	

Notes:

DATE: _____   S   M   T   W   T   F   S

Today Goals

Mood

- ○ Happy   ○ Stressed
- ○ Relaxed   ○ Anxious
- ○ Tired   ○ Sad
- ○ Inspired   ○ Angry

Energy Level

○	○	○
Low	Med	High

Blood Sugar & Food Tracker

Time/Meal	Blood Sugar Levels		Foods
	Before	After	
Wake-up Reading			
Breakfast			
Lunch			
Dinner			
Snacks			
Bedtime Reading			

Meds / Supplements

Water Intake

Activity

Sleep

Daily Schedule

Time	
5:00	
6:00	
7:00	
8:00	
9:00	
10:00	
11:00	
12:00	
13:00	
14:00	
15:00	
16:00	
17:00	
18:00	
19:00	
20:00	
21:00	
22:00	
23:00	

Notes: _____

_____

_____

_____

_____

DATE : _____   S   M   T   W   T   F   S

Today Goals

_____
_____
_____
_____
_____
_____
_____

Mood

○ Happy   ○ Stressed
○ Relaxed   ○ Anxious
○ Tired   ○ Sad
○ Inspired   ○ Angry

Energy Level

○   ○   ○
Low   Med   High

Blood Sugar & Food Tracker

Time/Meal	Blood Sugar Levels		Foods
	Before	After	
Wake-up Reading			
Breakfast			
Lunch			
Dinner			
Snacks			
Bedtime Reading			

Meds / Supplements

Water Intake

Activity

Sleep

Daily Schedule

Time	
5:00	
6:00	
7:00	
8:00	
9:00	
10:00	
11:00	
12:00	
13:00	
14:00	
15:00	
16:00	
17:00	
18:00	
19:00	
20:00	
21:00	
22:00	
23:00	

Notes:

DATE: _____   S M T W T F S

Today Goals

_____
_____
_____
_____
_____
_____

Mood

○ Happy   ○ Stressed
○ Relaxed   ○ Anxious
○ Tired   ○ Sad
○ Inspired   ○ Angry

Energy Level

○   ○   ○
Low   Med   High

Blood Sugar & Food Tracker

Time/Meal	Blood Sugar Levels		Foods
	Before	After	
Wake-up Reading			
Breakfast			
Lunch			
Dinner			
Snacks			
Bedtime Reading			

Meds / Supplements

Water Intake

Activity

Sleep

Daily Schedule

Time	
5:00	
6:00	
7:00	
8:00	
9:00	
10:00	
11:00	
12:00	
13:00	
14:00	
15:00	
16:00	
17:00	
18:00	
19:00	
20:00	
21:00	
22:00	
23:00	

Notes:

DATE: _____   S   M   T   W   T   F   S

Today Goals

_____

_____

_____

_____

_____

_____

Mood

- ○ Happy
- ○ Relaxed
- ○ Tired
- ○ Inspired
- ○ Stressed
- ○ Anxious
- ○ Sad
- ○ Angry

Energy Level

○	○	○
Low	Med	High

Blood Sugar & Food Tracker

Time/Meal	Blood Sugar Levels		Foods
	Before	After	
Wake-up Reading			
Breakfast			
Lunch			
Dinner			
Snacks			
Bedtime Reading			

Meds / Supplements

Water Intake

Activity

Sleep

Daily Schedule

Time	
5:00	
6:00	
7:00	
8:00	
9:00	
10:00	
11:00	
12:00	
13:00	
14:00	
15:00	
16:00	
17:00	
18:00	
19:00	
20:00	
21:00	
22:00	
23:00	

Notes:

DATE: _____   S   M   T   W   T   F   S

Today Goals

_____
_____
_____
_____
_____
_____

Mood

○ Happy   ○ Stressed
○ Relaxed   ○ Anxious
○ Tired   ○ Sad
○ Inspired   ○ Angry

Energy Level

○   ○   ○
Low   Med   High

Blood Sugar & Food Tracker

Time/Meal	Blood Sugar Levels		Foods
	Before	After	
Wake-up Reading			
Breakfast			
Lunch			
Dinner			
Snacks			
Bedtime Reading			

Meds / Supplements

Water Intake

Activity

Sleep

Daily Schedule

5:00	
6:00	
7:00	
8:00	
9:00	
10:00	
11:00	
12:00	
13:00	
14:00	
15:00	
16:00	
17:00	
18:00	
19:00	
20:00	
21:00	
22:00	
23:00	

Notes: _____
_____
_____
_____
_____

DATE : _____   S   M   T   W   T   F   S

Today Goals

_____
_____
_____
_____
_____
_____

Mood

○ Happy   ○ Stressed
○ Relaxed   ○ Anxious
○ Tired   ○ Sad
○ Inspired   ○ Angry

Energy Level

○   ○   ○
Low   Med   High

Blood Sugar & Food Tracker

Time/Meal	Blood Sugar Levels		Foods
	Before	After	
Wake-up Reading			
Breakfast			
Lunch			
Dinner			
Snacks			
Bedtime Reading			

Meds / Supplements

Water Intake

Activity

Sleep

Daily Schedule

5:00	
6:00	
7:00	
8:00	
9:00	
10:00	
11:00	
12:00	
13:00	
14:00	
15:00	
16:00	
17:00	
18:00	
19:00	
20:00	
21:00	
22:00	
23:00	

Notes:

DATE: _____   S M T W T F S

Today Goals

_____
_____
_____
_____
_____
_____

Mood

○ Happy   ○ Stressed
○ Relaxed   ○ Anxious
○ Tired   ○ Sad
○ Inspired   ○ Angry

Energy Level

○ Low   ○ Med   ○ High

Blood Sugar & Food Tracker

Time/Meal	Blood Sugar Levels		Foods
	Before	After	
Wake-up Reading			
Breakfast			
Lunch			
Dinner			
Snacks			
Bedtime Reading			

Meds / Supplements

Water Intake

Activity

Sleep

Daily Schedule

Time	
5:00	
6:00	
7:00	
8:00	
9:00	
10:00	
11:00	
12:00	
13:00	
14:00	
15:00	
16:00	
17:00	
18:00	
19:00	
20:00	
21:00	
22:00	
23:00	

Notes: _____
_____
_____
_____
_____

DATE: _____   S   M   T   W   T   F   S

Today Goals

_____
_____
_____
_____
_____

Mood

○ Happy   ○ Stressed
○ Relaxed   ○ Anxious
○ Tired   ○ Sad
○ Inspired   ○ Angry

Energy Level

○ Low   ○ Med   ○ High

Blood Sugar & Food Tracker

Time/Meal	Blood Sugar Levels		Foods
	Before	After	
Wake-up Reading			
Breakfast			
Lunch			
Dinner			
Snacks			
Bedtime Reading			

Meds/Supplements

Water Intake

Activity

Sleep

Daily Schedule

Time	
5:00	
6:00	
7:00	
8:00	
9:00	
10:00	
11:00	
12:00	
13:00	
14:00	
15:00	
16:00	
17:00	
18:00	
19:00	
20:00	
21:00	
22:00	
23:00	

Notes:

DATE : _____   S   M   T   W   T   F   S

Today Goals

_____
_____
_____
_____
_____
_____

Mood

○ Happy   ○ Stressed
○ Relaxed   ○ Anxious
○ Tired   ○ Sad
○ Inspired   ○ Angry

Energy Level

| ○ | ○ | ○ |
| Low | Med | High |

Blood Sugar & Food Tracker

Time/Meal	Blood Sugar Levels		Foods
	Before	After	
Wake-up Reading			
Breakfast			
Lunch			
Dinner			
Snacks			
Bedtime Reading			

Meds / Supplements

Water Intake

Activity

Sleep

Daily Schedule

Time	
5:00	
6:00	
7:00	
8:00	
9:00	
10:00	
11:00	
12:00	
13:00	
14:00	
15:00	
16:00	
17:00	
18:00	
19:00	
20:00	
21:00	
22:00	
23:00	

Notes:

DATE: _____   S M T W T F S

Today Goals

_____
_____
_____
_____
_____
_____

Mood

○ Happy   ○ Stressed
○ Relaxed   ○ Anxious
○ Tired   ○ Sad
○ Inspired   ○ Angry

Energy Level

○ Low   ○ Med   ○ High

Blood Sugar & Food Tracker

Time/Meal	Blood Sugar Levels		Foods
	Before	After	
Wake-up Reading			
Breakfast			
Lunch			
Dinner			
Snacks			
Bedtime Reading			

Meds / Supplements

Water Intake

Activity

Sleep

Daily Schedule

5:00	
6:00	
7:00	
8:00	
9:00	
10:00	
11:00	
12:00	
13:00	
14:00	
15:00	
16:00	
17:00	
18:00	
19:00	
20:00	
21:00	
22:00	
23:00	

Notes: _____

_____

_____

_____

_____

DATE: _____ S M T W T F S

Today Goals

_____
_____
_____
_____
_____
_____

Mood

○ Happy   ○ Stressed
○ Relaxed   ○ Anxious
○ Tired   ○ Sad
○ Inspired   ○ Angry

Energy Level

○   ○   ○
Low   Med   High

Blood Sugar & Food Tracker

Time/Meal	Blood Sugar Levels		Foods
	Before	After	
Wake-up Reading			
Breakfast			
Lunch			
Dinner			
Snacks			
Bedtime Reading			

Meds / Supplements

Water Intake

Activity

Sleep

Daily Schedule

5:00	
6:00	
7:00	
8:00	
9:00	
10:00	
11:00	
12:00	
13:00	
14:00	
15:00	
16:00	
17:00	
18:00	
19:00	
20:00	
21:00	
22:00	
23:00	

Notes: _____

_____

_____

_____

_____

DATE: _____   S   M   T   W   T   F   S

Today Goals

Mood

- ○ Happy   ○ Stressed
- ○ Relaxed   ○ Anxious
- ○ Tired   ○ Sad
- ○ Inspired   ○ Angry

Energy Level

○	○	○
Low	Med	High

Blood Sugar & Food Tracker

Time/Meal	Blood Sugar Levels		Foods
	Before	After	
Wake-up Reading			
Breakfast			
Lunch			
Dinner			
Snacks			
Bedtime Reading			

Meds / Supplements

Water Intake

Activity

Sleep

Daily Schedule

Time	
5:00	
6:00	
7:00	
8:00	
9:00	
10:00	
11:00	
12:00	
13:00	
14:00	
15:00	
16:00	
17:00	
18:00	
19:00	
20:00	
21:00	
22:00	
23:00	

Notes:

DATE: _____   S   M   T   W   T   F   S

Today Goals

_____

_____

_____

_____

_____

_____

Mood

- ○ Happy
- ○ Relaxed
- ○ Tired
- ○ Inspired
- ○ Stressed
- ○ Anxious
- ○ Sad
- ○ Angry

Energy Level

| ○ | ○ | ○ |
| Low | Med | High |

Blood Sugar & Food Tracker

Time/Meal	Blood Sugar Levels		Foods
	Before	After	
Wake-up Reading			
Breakfast			
Lunch			
Dinner			
Snacks			
Bedtime Reading			

Meds / Supplements

Water Intake

Activity

Sleep

Daily Schedule

Time	
5:00	
6:00	
7:00	
8:00	
9:00	
10:00	
11:00	
12:00	
13:00	
14:00	
15:00	
16:00	
17:00	
18:00	
19:00	
20:00	
21:00	
22:00	
23:00	

Notes: _____
_____
_____
_____
_____

DATE : _____   S   M   T   W   T   F   S

Today Goals

_____

_____

_____

_____

_____

_____

Mood

○ Happy   ○ Stressed

○ Relaxed   ○ Anxious

○ Tired   ○ Sad

○ Inspired   ○ Angry

Energy Level

○   ○   ○
Low   Med   High

Blood Sugar & Food Tracker

Time/Meal	Blood Sugar Levels		Foods
	Before	After	
Wake-up Reading			
Breakfast			
Lunch			
Dinner			
Snacks			
Bedtime Reading			

Meds / Supplements

Water Intake

Activity

Sleep

Daily Schedule

Time	
5:00	
6:00	
7:00	
8:00	
9:00	
10:00	
11:00	
12:00	
13:00	
14:00	
15:00	
16:00	
17:00	
18:00	
19:00	
20:00	
21:00	
22:00	
23:00	

Notes: _____
_____
_____
_____
_____

DATE: _____   S   M   T   W   T   F   S

᭬ Today Goals ᭬

_____

_____

_____

_____

_____

_____

᭬ Mood ᭬

○ Happy   ○ Stressed
○ Relaxed   ○ Anxious
○ Tired   ○ Sad
○ Inspired   ○ Angry

᭬ Energy Level ᭬

| ○ | ○ | ○ |
| Low | Med | High |

᭬ Blood Sugar & Food Tracker ᭬

Time/Meal	Blood Sugar Levels		Foods
	Before	After	
Wake-up Reading			
Breakfast			
Lunch			
Dinner			
Snacks			
Bedtime Reading			

Meds / Supplements

Water Intake

Activity

Sleep

Daily Schedule

5:00	
6:00	
7:00	
8:00	
9:00	
10:00	
11:00	
12:00	
13:00	
14:00	
15:00	
16:00	
17:00	
18:00	
19:00	
20:00	
21:00	
22:00	
23:00	

Notes: _____

_____

_____

_____

_____

DATE: _____　　　　S　M　T　W　T　F　S

Today Goals

_____
_____
_____
_____
_____
_____

Mood

○ Happy　　　○ Stressed
○ Relaxed　　○ Anxious
○ Tired　　　○ Sad
○ Inspired　　○ Angry

Energy Level

○　　　　○　　　　○
Low　　　Med　　　High

Blood Sugar & Food Tracker

Time/Meal	Blood Sugar Levels		Foods
	Before	After	
Wake-up Reading			
Breakfast			
Lunch			
Dinner			
Snacks			
Bedtime Reading			

Meds / Supplements

Water Intake

Activity

Sleep

Daily Schedule

Time	
5:00	
6:00	
7:00	
8:00	
9:00	
10:00	
11:00	
12:00	
13:00	
14:00	
15:00	
16:00	
17:00	
18:00	
19:00	
20:00	
21:00	
22:00	
23:00	

Notes:

DATE: _____   S M T W T F S

Today Goals

_____
_____
_____
_____
_____
_____

Mood

○ Happy   ○ Stressed
○ Relaxed   ○ Anxious
○ Tired   ○ Sad
○ Inspired   ○ Angry

Energy Level

○   ○   ○
Low   Med   High

Blood Sugar & Food Tracker

Time/Meal	Blood Sugar Levels		Foods
	Before	After	
Wake-up Reading			
Breakfast			
Lunch			
Dinner			
Snacks			
Bedtime Reading			

Meds / Supplements

Water Intake

Activity

Sleep

Daily Schedule

Time	
5:00	
6:00	
7:00	
8:00	
9:00	
10:00	
11:00	
12:00	
13:00	
14:00	
15:00	
16:00	
17:00	
18:00	
19:00	
20:00	
21:00	
22:00	
23:00	

Notes:

DATE : _____   S   M   T   W   T   F   S

Today Goals

Mood

- ○ Happy   ○ Stressed
- ○ Relaxed   ○ Anxious
- ○ Tired   ○ Sad
- ○ Inspired   ○ Angry

Energy Level

| ○ | ○ | ○ |
| Low | Med | High |

Blood Sugar & Food Tracker

Time/Meal	Blood Sugar Levels		Foods
	Before	After	
Wake-up Reading			
Breakfast			
Lunch			
Dinner			
Snacks			
Bedtime Reading			

Meds / Supplements

Water Intake

Activity

Sleep

Daily Schedule

Time	
5:00	
6:00	
7:00	
8:00	
9:00	
10:00	
11:00	
12:00	
13:00	
14:00	
15:00	
16:00	
17:00	
18:00	
19:00	
20:00	
21:00	
22:00	
23:00	

Notes:

DATE: _____   S M T W T F S

Today Goals

_____
_____
_____
_____
_____
_____

Mood

- ○ Happy
- ○ Relaxed
- ○ Tired
- ○ Inspired
- ○ Stressed
- ○ Anxious
- ○ Sad
- ○ Angry

Energy Level

○	○	○
Low	Med	High

Blood Sugar & Food Tracker

Time/Meal	Blood Sugar Levels		Foods
	Before	After	
Wake-up Reading			
Breakfast			
Lunch			
Dinner			
Snacks			
Bedtime Reading			

Meds / Supplements

Water Intake

Activity

Sleep

Daily Schedule

Time	
5:00	
6:00	
7:00	
8:00	
9:00	
10:00	
11:00	
12:00	
13:00	
14:00	
15:00	
16:00	
17:00	
18:00	
19:00	
20:00	
21:00	
22:00	
23:00	

Notes: _____

_____

_____

_____

_____

DATE: _____   S M T W T F S

Today Goals

_____
_____
_____
_____
_____
_____

Mood

○ Happy   ○ Stressed
○ Relaxed   ○ Anxious
○ Tired   ○ Sad
○ Inspired   ○ Angry

Energy Level

○ Low   ○ Med   ○ High

Blood Sugar & Food Tracker

Time/Meal	Blood Sugar Levels		Foods
	Before	After	
Wake-up Reading			
Breakfast			
Lunch			
Dinner			
Snacks			
Bedtime Reading			

Meds / Supplements

Water Intake

Activity

Sleep

Daily Schedule

Time	
5:00	
6:00	
7:00	
8:00	
9:00	
10:00	
11:00	
12:00	
13:00	
14:00	
15:00	
16:00	
17:00	
18:00	
19:00	
20:00	
21:00	
22:00	
23:00	

Notes:

DATE : _____   S   M   T   W   T   F   S

Today Goals

_____

_____

_____

_____

_____

_____

Mood

○ Happy   ○ Stressed

○ Relaxed   ○ Anxious

○ Tired   ○ Sad

○ Inspired   ○ Angry

Energy Level

○   ○   ○
Low   Med   High

Blood Sugar & Food Tracker

Time/Meal	Blood Sugar Levels		Foods
	Before	After	
Wake-up Reading			
Breakfast			
Lunch			
Dinner			
Snacks			
Bedtime Reading			

Meds / Supplements

Water Intake

Activity

Sleep

Daily Schedule

Time	
5:00	
6:00	
7:00	
8:00	
9:00	
10:00	
11:00	
12:00	
13:00	
14:00	
15:00	
16:00	
17:00	
18:00	
19:00	
20:00	
21:00	
22:00	
23:00	

Notes:

DATE: _____ S M T W T F S

Today Goals

_____

_____

_____

_____

_____

_____

Mood

○ Happy   ○ Stressed
○ Relaxed   ○ Anxious
○ Tired   ○ Sad
○ Inspired   ○ Angry

Energy Level

○   ○   ○
Low   Med   High

Blood Sugar & Food Tracker

Time/Meal	Blood Sugar Levels		Foods
	Before	After	
Wake-up Reading			
Breakfast			
Lunch			
Dinner			
Snacks			
Bedtime Reading			

Meds / Supplements

Water Intake

Activity

Sleep

Daily Schedule

5:00	
6:00	
7:00	
8:00	
9:00	
10:00	
11:00	
12:00	
13:00	
14:00	
15:00	
16:00	
17:00	
18:00	
19:00	
20:00	
21:00	
22:00	
23:00	

Notes: _____

_____

_____

_____

_____

DATE : _____   S M T W T F S

Today Goals

_____
_____
_____
_____
_____
_____

Mood

○ Happy   ○ Stressed
○ Relaxed   ○ Anxious
○ Tired   ○ Sad
○ Inspired   ○ Angry

Energy Level

○   ○   ○
Low   Med   High

Blood Sugar & Food Tracker

Time/Meal	Blood Sugar Levels		Foods
	Before	After	
Wake-up Reading			
Breakfast			
Lunch			
Dinner			
Snacks			
Bedtime Reading			

Meds / Supplements

Water Intake

Activity

Sleep

Daily Schedule

Time	
5:00	
6:00	
7:00	
8:00	
9:00	
10:00	
11:00	
12:00	
13:00	
14:00	
15:00	
16:00	
17:00	
18:00	
19:00	
20:00	
21:00	
22:00	
23:00	

Notes:

DATE : _____   S   M   T   W   T   F   S

Today Goals

_____
_____
_____
_____
_____
_____
_____

Mood

○ Happy   ○ Stressed
○ Relaxed   ○ Anxious
○ Tired   ○ Sad
○ Inspired   ○ Angry

Energy Level

| ○ | ○ | ○ |
| Low | Med | High |

Blood Sugar & Food Tracker

Time/Meal	Blood Sugar Levels		Foods
	Before	After	
Wake-up Reading			
Breakfast			
Lunch			
Dinner			
Snacks			
Bedtime Reading			

Meds / Supplements

Water Intake

Activity

Sleep

Daily Schedule

5:00	
6:00	
7:00	
8:00	
9:00	
10:00	
11:00	
12:00	
13:00	
14:00	
15:00	
16:00	
17:00	
18:00	
19:00	
20:00	
21:00	
22:00	
23:00	

Notes: _____

_____

_____

_____

_____

DATE: _____   S M T W T F S

Today Goals

_____

_____

_____

_____

_____

_____

Mood

- ○ Happy
- ○ Relaxed
- ○ Tired
- ○ Inspired
- ○ Stressed
- ○ Anxious
- ○ Sad
- ○ Angry

Energy Level

○	○	○
Low	Med	High

Blood Sugar & Food Tracker

Time/Meal	Blood Sugar Levels		Foods
	Before	After	
Wake-up Reading			
Breakfast			
Lunch			
Dinner			
Snacks			
Bedtime Reading			

Meds / Supplements

Water Intake

Activity

Sleep

Daily Schedule

Time	
5:00	
6:00	
7:00	
8:00	
9:00	
10:00	
11:00	
12:00	
13:00	
14:00	
15:00	
16:00	
17:00	
18:00	
19:00	
20:00	
21:00	
22:00	
23:00	

Notes: _____
_____
_____
_____
_____

DATE: _____   S M T W T F S

Today Goals

_____
_____
_____
_____
_____
_____

Mood

○ Happy   ○ Stressed
○ Relaxed   ○ Anxious
○ Tired   ○ Sad
○ Inspired   ○ Angry

Energy Level

○   ○   ○
Low   Med   High

Blood Sugar & Food Tracker

Time/Meal	Blood Sugar Levels		Foods
	Before	After	
Wake-up Reading			
Breakfast			
Lunch			
Dinner			
Snacks			
Bedtime Reading			

Meds / Supplements

Water Intake

Activity

Sleep

Daily Schedule

Time	
5:00	
6:00	
7:00	
8:00	
9:00	
10:00	
11:00	
12:00	
13:00	
14:00	
15:00	
16:00	
17:00	
18:00	
19:00	
20:00	
21:00	
22:00	
23:00	

Notes: _____

_____

_____

_____

_____

DATE : _____   S   M   T   W   T   F   S

Today Goals

_____

_____

_____

_____

_____

_____

Mood

○ Happy	○ Stressed
○ Relaxed	○ Anxious
○ Tired	○ Sad
○ Inspired	○ Angry

Energy Level

○	○	○
Low	Med	High

Blood Sugar & Food Tracker

Time/Meal	Blood Sugar Levels		Foods
	Before	After	
Wake-up Reading			
Breakfast			
Lunch			
Dinner			
Snacks			
Bedtime Reading			

Meds / Supplements

Water Intake

Activity

Sleep

Daily Schedule

Time	
5:00	
6:00	
7:00	
8:00	
9:00	
10:00	
11:00	
12:00	
13:00	
14:00	
15:00	
16:00	
17:00	
18:00	
19:00	
20:00	
21:00	
22:00	
23:00	

Notes:

DATE: _____   S M T W T F S

Today Goals

_____
_____
_____
_____
_____
_____

Mood

- ○ Happy
- ○ Relaxed
- ○ Tired
- ○ Inspired
- ○ Stressed
- ○ Anxious
- ○ Sad
- ○ Angry

Energy Level

○	○	○
Low	Med	High

Blood Sugar & Food Tracker

Time/Meal	Blood Sugar Levels		Foods
	Before	After	
Wake-up Reading			
Breakfast			
Lunch			
Dinner			
Snacks			
Bedtime Reading			

Meds / Supplements

Water Intake

Activity

Sleep

Daily Schedule

5:00	
6:00	
7:00	
8:00	
9:00	
10:00	
11:00	
12:00	
13:00	
14:00	
15:00	
16:00	
17:00	
18:00	
19:00	
20:00	
21:00	
22:00	
23:00	

Notes: _____

_____

_____

_____

_____

Today Goals

_____
_____
_____
_____
_____
_____

Mood

- ○ Happy   ○ Stressed
- ○ Relaxed   ○ Anxious
- ○ Tired   ○ Sad
- ○ Inspired   ○ Angry

Energy Level

○	○	○
Low	Med	High

Blood Sugar & Food Tracker

Time/Meal	Blood Sugar Levels		Foods
	Before	After	
Wake-up Reading			
Breakfast			
Lunch			
Dinner			
Snacks			
Bedtime Reading			

Meds / Supplements

Water Intake

Activity

Sleep

Daily Schedule

Time	
5:00	
6:00	
7:00	
8:00	
9:00	
10:00	
11:00	
12:00	
13:00	
14:00	
15:00	
16:00	
17:00	
18:00	
19:00	
20:00	
21:00	
22:00	
23:00	

Notes:

_____

_____

_____

_____

_____

DATE : _____   S   M   T   W   T   F   S

Today Goals

_____
_____
_____
_____
_____
_____

Mood

○ Happy   ○ Stressed
○ Relaxed   ○ Anxious
○ Tired   ○ Sad
○ Inspired   ○ Angry

Energy Level

○	○	○
Low	Med	High

Blood Sugar & Food Tracker

Time/Meal	Blood Sugar Levels		Foods
	Before	After	
Wake-up Reading			
Breakfast			
Lunch			
Dinner			
Snacks			
Bedtime Reading			

Meds / Supplements

Water Intake

Activity

Sleep

Daily Schedule

Time	
5:00	
6:00	
7:00	
8:00	
9:00	
10:00	
11:00	
12:00	
13:00	
14:00	
15:00	
16:00	
17:00	
18:00	
19:00	
20:00	
21:00	
22:00	
23:00	

Notes:

DATE : _____   S M T W T F S

Today Goals

_____
_____
_____
_____
_____
_____

Mood

- ○ Happy   ○ Stressed
- ○ Relaxed   ○ Anxious
- ○ Tired   ○ Sad
- ○ Inspired   ○ Angry

Energy Level

○	○	○
Low	Med	High

Blood Sugar & Food Tracker

Time/Meal	Blood Sugar Levels		Foods
	Before	After	
Wake-up Reading			
Breakfast			
Lunch			
Dinner			
Snacks			
Bedtime Reading			

Meds / Supplements

Water Intake

Activity

Sleep

Daily Schedule

Time	
5:00	
6:00	
7:00	
8:00	
9:00	
10:00	
11:00	
12:00	
13:00	
14:00	
15:00	
16:00	
17:00	
18:00	
19:00	
20:00	
21:00	
22:00	
23:00	

Notes: _____

_____

_____

_____

_____

DATE: _____   S M T W T F S

Today Goals

_____

_____

_____

_____

_____

Mood

○ Happy   ○ Stressed

○ Relaxed   ○ Anxious

○ Tired   ○ Sad

○ Inspired   ○ Angry

Energy Level

○ Low   ○ Med   ○ High

Blood Sugar & Food Tracker

Time/Meal	Blood Sugar Levels		Foods
	Before	After	
Wake-up Reading			
Breakfast			
Lunch			
Dinner			
Snacks			
Bedtime Reading			

Meds / Supplements

Water Intake

Activity

Sleep

Daily Schedule

Time	
5:00	
6:00	
7:00	
8:00	
9:00	
10:00	
11:00	
12:00	
13:00	
14:00	
15:00	
16:00	
17:00	
18:00	
19:00	
20:00	
21:00	
22:00	
23:00	

Notes: _____
_____
_____
_____
_____

DATE : _____   S M T W T F S

Today Goals

_____
_____
_____
_____
_____
_____

Mood

○ Happy   ○ Stressed
○ Relaxed   ○ Anxious
○ Tired   ○ Sad
○ Inspired   ○ Angry

Energy Level

○   ○   ○
Low   Med   High

Blood Sugar & Food Tracker

Time/Meal	Blood Sugar Levels		Foods
	Before	After	
Wake-up Reading			
Breakfast			
Lunch			
Dinner			
Snacks			
Bedtime Reading			

Meds / Supplements

Water Intake

Activity

Sleep

Daily Schedule

Time	
5:00	
6:00	
7:00	
8:00	
9:00	
10:00	
11:00	
12:00	
13:00	
14:00	
15:00	
16:00	
17:00	
18:00	
19:00	
20:00	
21:00	
22:00	
23:00	

Notes:

DATE: _____   S M T W T F S

Today Goals

_____
_____
_____
_____
_____
_____

Mood

○ Happy   ○ Stressed
○ Relaxed   ○ Anxious
○ Tired   ○ Sad
○ Inspired   ○ Angry

Energy Level

○   ○   ○
Low   Med   High

Blood Sugar & Food Tracker

Time/Meal	Blood Sugar Levels		Foods
	Before	After	
Wake-up Reading			
Breakfast			
Lunch			
Dinner			
Snacks			
Bedtime Reading			

Meds / Supplements

Water Intake

Activity

Sleep

Daily Schedule

5:00	
6:00	
7:00	
8:00	
9:00	
10:00	
11:00	
12:00	
13:00	
14:00	
15:00	
16:00	
17:00	
18:00	
19:00	
20:00	
21:00	
22:00	
23:00	

Notes:

DATE: _____   S M T W T F S

Today Goals

_____
_____
_____
_____
_____
_____

Mood

○ Happy   ○ Stressed
○ Relaxed   ○ Anxious
○ Tired   ○ Sad
○ Inspired   ○ Angry

Energy Level

○   ○   ○
Low   Med   High

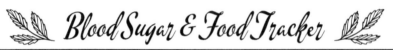

Blood Sugar & Food Tracker

Time/Meal	Blood Sugar Levels		Foods
	Before	After	
Wake-up Reading			
Breakfast			
Lunch			
Dinner			
Snacks			
Bedtime Reading			

Meds/Supplements

Water Intake

Activity

Sleep

Daily Schedule

Time	
5:00	
6:00	
7:00	
8:00	
9:00	
10:00	
11:00	
12:00	
13:00	
14:00	
15:00	
16:00	
17:00	
18:00	
19:00	
20:00	
21:00	
22:00	
23:00	

Notes: _____

_____

_____

_____

_____

DATE : _____   S   M   T   W   T   F   S

Today Goals

_____

_____

_____

_____

_____

_____

Mood

○ Happy   ○ Stressed

○ Relaxed   ○ Anxious

○ Tired   ○ Sad

○ Inspired   ○ Angry

Energy Level

○ Low   ○ Med   ○ High

Blood Sugar & Food Tracker

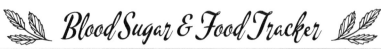

Time/Meal	Blood Sugar Levels		Foods
	Before	After	
Wake-up Reading			
Breakfast			
Lunch			
Dinner			
Snacks			
Bedtime Reading			

Meds / Supplements

Water Intake

Activity

Sleep

Daily Schedule

5:00	
6:00	
7:00	
8:00	
9:00	
10:00	
11:00	
12:00	
13:00	
14:00	
15:00	
16:00	
17:00	
18:00	
19:00	
20:00	
21:00	
22:00	
23:00	

Notes:

DATE: _____   S   M   T   W   T   F   S

Today Goals

_____

_____

_____

_____

_____

Mood

○ Happy   ○ Stressed

○ Relaxed   ○ Anxious

○ Tired   ○ Sad

○ Inspired   ○ Angry

Energy Level

○ Low   ○ Med   ○ High

Blood Sugar & Food Tracker

Time/Meal	Blood Sugar Levels		Foods
	Before	After	
Wake-up Reading			
Breakfast			
Lunch			
Dinner			
Snacks			
Bedtime Reading			

Meds / Supplements

Water Intake

Activity

Sleep

Daily Schedule

Time	
5:00	
6:00	
7:00	
8:00	
9:00	
10:00	
11:00	
12:00	
13:00	
14:00	
15:00	
16:00	
17:00	
18:00	
19:00	
20:00	
21:00	
22:00	
23:00	

Notes: _____

_____

_____

_____

_____

DATE: _____   S M T W T F S

Today Goals

_____
_____
_____
_____
_____
_____

Mood

○ Happy   ○ Stressed
○ Relaxed   ○ Anxious
○ Tired   ○ Sad
○ Inspired   ○ Angry

Energy Level

○	○	○
Low	Med	High

Blood Sugar & Food Tracker

Time/Meal	Blood Sugar Levels		Foods
	Before	After	
Wake-up Reading			
Breakfast			
Lunch			
Dinner			
Snacks			
Bedtime Reading			

Meds / Supplements

Water Intake

Activity

Sleep

Daily Schedule

Time	
5:00	
6:00	
7:00	
8:00	
9:00	
10:00	
11:00	
12:00	
13:00	
14:00	
15:00	
16:00	
17:00	
18:00	
19:00	
20:00	
21:00	
22:00	
23:00	

Notes: _____

_____

_____

_____

_____

DATE : _____   S M T W T F S

Today Goals

_____
_____
_____
_____
_____
_____
_____

Mood

○ Happy   ○ Stressed
○ Relaxed   ○ Anxious
○ Tired   ○ Sad
○ Inspired   ○ Angry

Energy Level

○   ○   ○
Low   Med   High

Blood Sugar & Food Tracker

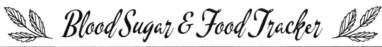

Time/Meal	Blood Sugar Levels		Foods
	Before	After	
Wake-up Reading			
Breakfast			
Lunch			
Dinner			
Snacks			
Bedtime Reading			

Printed in Great Britain
by Amazon

43992751R00069